I0792331

Genes and Chromosomes

in Cancer

Dr Judy Ford B.Sc. (Hons), Ph.D.

About the author

Judy Ford PhD is a geneticist, who worked in Human Cytogenetics from the early years when chromosome analysis was very new, and DNA analysis was in its infancy.

She started her work in Cancer Research in 1969 at the Karolinska Institute, which was then located at Sydney Hospital. She then moved to Adelaide where she was invited to set up a Cytogenetics Laboratory at The Queen Elizabeth Hospital, a Teaching Hospital of the University of Adelaide. She led this laboratory until 1995 when the South Australian Government centralised all laboratory services. Judy then set up a private laboratory (GCAT) Genetic Consulting & Testing, which closed in 2000 due to vested interests who targeted her laboratory because they didn't want people to know that chemical exposures were causing cancer!

Dr Judy's work involved many different aspects of Genetics. In all she published about 100 scientific papers that are listed in Google Scholar. Of these, 14 are specifically concerned with cancer and another 17 are concerned with the cellular mechanisms that underlie chromosomal error. This makes her unusual in having had a long-term interest in studying the cellular conditions and environmental and lifestyle factors that underlie cancer.

Table of Contents

Chapter One

What is Cancer?   5

Chapter Two

How does a Normal Cell become a Cancer Cell?   25

Chapter Three

Genes that confer susceptibility to Cancer   55

Chapter Four

Changes in DNA and Chromosomes that cause Cancer   64

Chapter Five

Epigenetics – yet another layer of complexity   95

References   107

Chapter One

What is a Cancer?

Cancer is the name given to any *invasive growth* in *any organism* that is caused by abnormal and uncontrolled cell division. Almost all cells that become cancerous, start their life as completely normal cells!

Cancer can affect many organisms, including lower organisms like invertebrates, and is not limited to humans and larger, longer-lived organisms:

Invertebrates

Cancers have been reported in many invertebrates including aquatic species such as corals and jellyfish, and worms of all types.

Crustacea such as shrimp can develop tumours that resemble lymphomas. These seem to be associated with viral infections and can lead to both abnormal growth and metastases (i.e. they can spread from the initial location in the body to other locations).

Multicellular organisms

Cancer can be found in some 'individuals' in all types of multicellular organisms including plants, fungi, algae, and metazoans.

Animals

Cancer is widespread throughout the animal kingdom. It affects molluscs, fish, reptiles, birds, and all mammals. Some species develop cancers that are very similar to humans, while others are affected by much rarer specific and contagious forms of the disease.

Cancer Initiation

In most if not all cancers, the cancer starts in <u>one location in the body</u> and is usually initiated in just one cell or at most a small group of cells.

In mammals, many cells that have the potential to become cancers are destroyed by a healthy immune system, so for most people, cancer prevention requires **both** avoiding carcinogens (cancer causing agents) and strengthening the immune and defence systems.

Very importantly, since stress suppresses immune systems, avoiding stress is critical to staying healthy.

Is a tumour the same as a cancer?

There is a subtle but important difference, and the two terms are often confused or interchanged.

However, a tumour is an abnormal lump composed of cells that have grown quickly and have lost many of their proper controls. A tumour can become a cancer, but many tumours remain harmless lumps. Nevertheless, if a tumour cell undergoes changes that allow it to overcome the body's normal control mechanisms, it is now a cancer and it may spread to other parts of the body through the lymphatic system or the blood stream. It is very important that all tumours are thoroughly investigated and treated appropriately.

Naming Cancers

The names that have been given to the various cancers usually describe either the organ or tissue in which the cancer resides (e.g. liver cancer), or the type of cell from which the cancer grew (e.g. megaloblastic leukemia), but occasionally cancers are known by the name of the person who discovered them (e.g. Burkitt's lymphoma).

These differences in *naming* the cancers can be confusing, but they are mostly irrelevant to us, provided we realise that they are all cancers and so, behave in a similar way.

Every different type of cancer has its own specific characteristics and prognosis. For example, pancreatic cancer is largely incurable - 80% of patients die within one year - whereas prostate cancer patients have a 95% chance of living for at least five years or more after their diagnosis.

The burden of cancer has been vastly increased by modern environments, lifestyle, AND world overpopulation

Overpopulation, destruction of natural environments and cancer

Although there are a few cancers that are caused by inherited gene abnormalities or spontaneous mistakes in DNA replication or cell division, most cancers are caused by external agents. These are usually infectious agents and/or toxic environmental chemicals. Both types of carcinogens are now much more prevalent throughout the world because of overpopulation, destruction of natural environments, as well as current and past manufacturing and agricultural practices, and modern lifestyles.

The concept of zero population growth (ZPG) was a popular movement in the 1960s when many thoughtful people recognized that, as the world continued to '*save people from death* through various humanitarian acts, we should equally limit reproduction.

Paul Ehrlich, the author of The Population Bomb[1] stated that "The mother of the year should be a sterile woman with two adopted children". However, in contrast to this advice, most modern economies are constructed to depend on continuous growth and such growth necessitates destruction of the environment as well as causing ever-increasing rates of cancer.

Whatever our personal views of ZPG, it is easy to see that many populations of people who live in areas where there is naturally high childhood mortality compensate by having larger numbers of children. Such high fertility improves the likelihood that threatened populations are sustained.

However, if as commonly occurs, various 'groups' intervene to reduce the effects of childhood mortality, without also introducing contraception, massive population growth ensues. Sadly, just 'doing good' can inadvertently cause bigger problems! But this is just an introduction to this massive world problem, which will not be discussed further here.

Some of the consequences of over-population that have directly contributed to cancer are:

<u>The destruction of the natural habitats of a variety of animals</u> has brought animals and the various microorganisms they carry into closer proximity with humans. This is also thought to be the cause of the disease pandemics that currently affect the world.

<u>The overuse of land (both in size and intensity) for agriculture</u> has necessitated enormous use of herbicides and insecticides. It has also caused a huge reduction of minerals and other soil nutrients. Normal soil microbiota is vastly changed by both overuse and chemicals.

The introduction and expansive growth of manufactured food has led to reduced ingestion of natural nutrients and the introduction of a immense range of chemicals into food.

Mining, manufacturing, and deforestation have all caused general destruction of natural environments and have led to vast pollution of air and water with worldwide consequences such as climate change.

Local pollution of soil and water has directly increased cancer risks in the communities living nearby.

Light pollution of night skies has caused disruptions of normal daily rhythms and individual people's melatonin production. In turn, this has resulted in both physical and mental health issues as well as possibly being 'carcinogenic'.

This disruption of diurnal rhythms is further exacerbated in people who work in night shifts. Long-term shiftwork for 19 months or more has been reported to increase cancer risk by up to 20%.

<u>Stresses</u> from many different aspects of modern life, including the breakdown of relationships, has major effects on health. Stress suppresses the immune system and as well as reducing resistance to infectious agents, allows cancers to grow!

<u>Economic policies that depend on continuous industry and population growth for 'success'</u>, are also (inadvertently) major contributors to the increasing burden of cancer.

What are the direct causes of cancer?

Although there are some inherited genes that influence about 5 – 10% of the population's susceptibility to cancer, and a small number of people have greatly elevated risks due to other aspects of their genetic constitution, most causes of cancer are found in lifestyle and environment. This is undisputed.

There are many different lines of evidence that prove that environmental exposures are the primary cause of cancer but the different rates of cancers in dissimilar societies give us valuable insight into the causes. Furthermore, since most individuals' cancer risks change when they move from one country or 'area' to another, we can be sure that environmental and lifestyle exposures and behaviours are the key factors in most cancers.

Although many diverse factors cause cancer, many of the factors can be grouped. These include:

- *Infectious agents*, especially viruses, and sometimes a cancer is caused by one infectious agent working with another. Alternatively, we see that an infection might function with a food or chemical to cause cancer.

  For example, infection by the ubiquitous *Epstein Barr Virus* (EBV – a herpes virus) causes an illness known as *glandular fever in people* who contract it in adolescence or adulthood. The symptoms may be quite severe and prolonged, or a mild and quite short illness, but once infected, EBV usually stays in a person's body. Many people are infected by EBV as children and often have no obvious symptoms. Nevertheless, at least 90% of the world's population has been infected by EBV.

If a person who carries EBV is exposed to Malaria, they have a relatively high chance of developing *Burkitt's Lymphoma.* Malaria itself is usually caused by the unicellular, protozoan *Plasmodium falciparum* (or one of three other Plasmodia).

EBV is also strongly 'associated' with *Hodgkin's Lymphoma* as well as with *Stomach Cancer* and *Breast Cancer*. The medical literature shows that EBV is present in most of the tumours examined and it seems to play an active role in the disease process.

At the time of writing, there is no doubt that EBV is activated in all the cancers named above and possibly in many others, but its function in the development and progression of different tumours is still not sufficiently well understood.

- *Radiation – including X-rays, radon, and UV light.* Each of these forms of radiation can cause cancer but in different ways. X-Rays break chromosomes in an apparently random manner. Radon is radioactive but it decays very quickly and as it decays it releases small radioactive particles that damage the cells in the lung. Hence, Radon is specifically associated with lung cancer. UV light causes thymidine dimers and will be discussed in a later section.

- *Chemical carcinogens* – including tobacco, asbestos, DDT and many other insecticides and herbicides.

  The 2021 USA National Toxicology program currently lists 256 substances - chemical, physical, and biological agents; mixtures; and exposure circumstances - that are known or reasonably anticipated to cause cancer in humans.

- *Diet and lifestyle* – Many of these exposures are included in the 256 substances mentioned above. In other words, normal, daily life in a modern society will expose you to many carcinogens unless you are extraordinarily vigilant.

Different Composition of Cancers in different Countries

Several international organisations independently collect data on cancer incidences. Some data sets report the rates of cancer diagnoses and others report the rates of cancer deaths. Unfortunately, the different data sets do not necessarily include all the same countries because of varied availability of information. There is also some inconsistency between data sets that (probably) reflects differences in the accuracy of the reporting systems and/or the time of data collection.

Despite these limitations, the data is reasonably sound and can be used to give us valuable insight into the causes of most cancers.

Australia, where I live, has the highest overall incidence of cancers partly because of its exceptionally high rate of skin cancer. However, while Australia's score is high for several different cancers, its rate of early diagnosis and intervention is also high. This results in lower death rates in Australia from some cancers that are lethal in many countries with less accessible healthcare.

Unfortunately, the high 'cure rate' gives Australians (and others who live in 'like' countries) a false sense that people are healthier than they are!

The Effect of Globalisation on Cancer Rates

Change in cultures and exposures caused by global trade cause changes in cancer rates. This is shown dramatically in Japan where a 'western' culture was imported after the second world war and many traditional foods and cultural practices were reduced.

The following graph shows that since 1975 breast cancer in Japan has approximately doubled at all ages from about 32 to 80. Above 80, there is an increase, but it is not as dramatic. Below age 32, breast cancer is rare, and as in Australia is mostly caused by inherited factors rather than environmental. In contrast, above about age 32, the causes are mostly environmental although there are many genes that can affect risk.

The reduced change observed in this graph in those aged 80 and older possibly reflects the far lower tendency of older persons to change their lifestyle. However, it may also reflect the ages at which exposures are important.

Figure: Change in rates of Breast Cancer by Age in Japanese women from 1975 to 1996

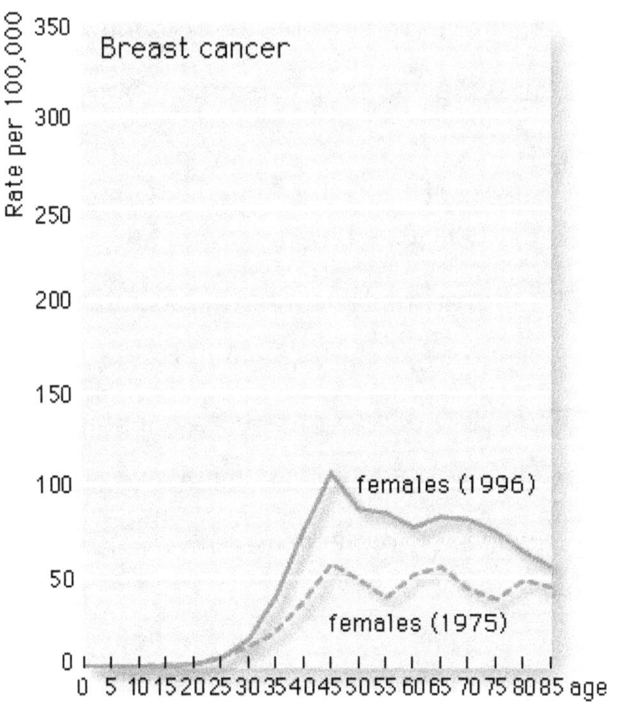

Summary

Most people are aware that there are environmental and lifestyle factors that influence the risk of some cancers. Most are aware of the association between cigarette smoking and lung cancer and of sunburn and skin cancer.

Perhaps what is less well understood, however, is that almost all the world's cancer burden is related to lifestyle and environment and could be prevented. The differences in cancer rates between places, between cultures and between changes in culture, prove this causal relationship.

Chapter Two

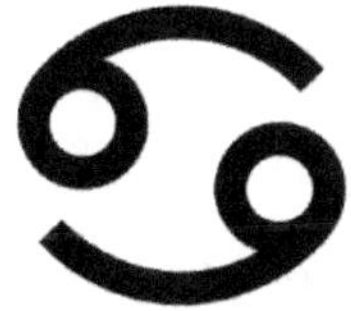

How does a Normal Cell become a Cancer Cell?

Starting at the beginning

Before defining a cancer cell, we need to describe normal cells because normal cells vary a great deal so that they can perform their diverse functions.

Definition: Normal Human Cell

A normal cell has the following characteristics:

1. Each cell has a specific function.
2. Each cell is usually part of lineage of cells whose function has been set during early embryonic development.
3. Each cell has *specific shape* and *sub-cellular architecture*.
4. With the exception of 'stem cells', and the reproductive cells that produce sperm, all other cells have a strictly pre-defined limit of cell divisions.
5. With *only* the exception of mature red blood cells, all other cells have a nucleus that contains DNA. Moreover, almost all cells (and again

except sperm), have the DNA content of 46 chromosomes including one pair of sex chromosomes and one pair of each of the 22 autosomes. In each (normal) case, the DNA of one of the chromosome pair will have been maternally derived and one paternally derived.

6. All cells contain organelles (small, discrete functional units) but the mitochondria, which are also absent from red blood cells, are maternally inherited in the oocyte (egg) cytoplasm. The male's mitochondria are *not* passed on to his offspring.

Mitochondria are responsible for the generation of energy in the cell. They are thought to have arisen from some ancestral bacteria or bacteria-like organism that was incorporated into the cells of primitive organisms to provide a system of generating energy.

7. The division of a normal cell *within an organ or tissue* is strictly limited by the normal boundaries of other cells.

8. The division of a normal cell is strictly controlled by several signalling pathways.

9. Each normal cell is subject to seek and destroy mechanisms that are in place to eliminate defects and keep the organism in good condition.

The Evolution of a Cancer Cell

Cancer usually occurs from the accumulation of several or even many changes that each alter one of the characteristics of a normal cell. The cell might still retain some of the characteristics of the cell lineage from which it was initiated but invasive cancer cells no longer have any of the normal controls.

All changes that occur in cancer cells involve changes in the function of individual genes. Some genes have especially important regulatory functions, and these genes are altered in many cancers. Such genes are usually classified as tumour suppressor genes because their normal function is to reduce or control cell division and they may promote apoptosis (programmed cell death).

The *p53 gene* is one such important gene and possibly the most important!

The first stage in the evolution of a cancer cell is usually called MUTATION, the second is called PROMOTION and the third is called PROGRESSION.

At the end of its evolution, a cancer cell has lost all the normal constraints of a normal cell. Not only can it divide continuously it can climb over other cells and generally behave like an exceptionally bad and intrusive neighbour!

Some tumours invade other tissues to form what are called secondary tumours or masses in other tissues and organs in different parts of the body. The cancer cells usually move into these secondary areas through the *blood* or *lymph circulatory systems*. For this reason, it is essential for doctors who are treating cancer patients to look for the possible presence of cancer cells in lymph glands near the original tumour.

Angiogenesis is the ability of a tumour to induce the formation of new blood vessels. Once a tumour has developed this ability, it is able to set up its own blood supply to feed its own growth of abnormal cells. Angiogenesis usually occurs at an advanced stage of malignancy.

Cancer Progression

Stage 1 - Mutation

The general term MUTATION describes a change in a gene. This usually means that the DNA or code of the gene is changed. However, there can sometimes be a change in the function of a gene without a change to the actual DNA and this type of change, usually called an *epigenetic* change can also occur in cancer.

The following is a list of the types of genetic change that commonly occur in cancer cells. I will describe each in more detail later. The changes are:

Single gene mutation: An alteration occurs in the genetic code of a single gene. Cancer generating mutations change a critical regulatory function.

Chromosomal break: A break occurs in the structure of a chromosome. This can have several consequences, and most breaks generate dramatic changes in one or more genes (often many genes) and their function.

Polyploidy: If a cell fails to complete cell division after the DNA has been replicated, then the cell will have double (or more in some cases) the normal number of chromosomes. This cell might not cause too many problems unless it attempts to undergo further cell division, but further cell division is then likely to be highly error prone and generate many abnormal 'daughter' cells. This type of division is extremely common in 'solid' tumours.

Epigenetic change in gene function: A change in the function of a gene or regulation of a gene may be caused by other factors other than a change in the DNA itself. So-called epigenetic changes often involve modifications of the proteins that associate with DNA and are involved in the translation of genetic information.

Stage 2 - Promotion

Uncontrolled cell division is one of the essential features of cancer, *but* it is normal cell division that creates opportunities for cancer to emerge. It is important to understand this as most cancer texts fail to emphasise this.

On any occasion when a cell divides, there is an opportunity for a MUTATION to be promoted. So, to reduce our cancer risk, we must aim to keep our rate of cell division to a minimum. This will also reduce our rate of ageing!

Although reducing cell divisions is probably easier said than done, I will suggest some approaches we might take.

During foetal development there are masses of cells dividing. During growth from baby to adult, there are masses of cells dividing. Throughout our lifespan cells divide to maintain the structure and function of our organs and tissues. Every one of these cell divisions theoretically provides an opportunity for a cancer to emerge.

Damage to a gene or chromosome is of no consequence until the cell goes through the next round of DNA replication in preparation for cell division. Although the damage is converted into a mutation at the time of DNA synthesis, it is still unlikely to cause a problem unless the cell itself divides! However, when the cell does divide, two abnormal cells will be created and there will be more opportunity for the expression of a dangerous gene.

Here is a short list of some of the occasions of excessive cell division that *can* be avoided:

- Sunburn. This may be the easiest. Either cover up and/or use protective sunscreen, especially if you live in Australia, where we have the highest rates of skin cancer in the world.

- Cuts and Abrasions particularly from large accidents are a major occasion of excess cell divisions. Take care and wherever possible use protective gloves and clothing. If you are older, undertake strengthening exercises to minimise your risks of falling and don't be too proud to use equipment that will minimise the risks of falling.

- Operations - all *unnecessary* medical operations should be avoided and where possible less invasive forms of surgery should be chosen!

- Infections. Do what you can to avoid all contagious infections. When they are sick, young children are much more contagious than adults because their immune systems are immature.

  Two key factors that influence the duration of viral shedding are age and severity of illness. Young children, because of their relative lack of immunity, can shed virus for 10 days or more. Patients with chronic diseases and more severe, complicated influenza shed the virus for an average of 2 days longer than uncomplicated influenza. In elderly and immunocompromised patients, viral shedding and potential infectivity can persist for weeks, even months. [i]

- To make sure you protect yourself, always wear a mask when near a sick person and insist on everyone having 'clean hands.

To illustrate what is required with 'clean hands' I refer to an occasion years ago when I worked in a hospital. We had an 'open day' and to demonstrate the effect of good hand washing, staff from the Microbiology Department asked everyone to place their unwashed hands on a petri dish and then go and wash their hands. On their return they were asked to touch a second dish with their now 'supposedly' clean hands. The idea was to show that hand washing reduced bacteria!

So, I took my two young children and was bemused when their agar plates showed much greater contamination after their inadequate hand washing than their initial dry dirty hands!

My own hands were clean – a result of excellent hand cleaning techniques developed during working with tissue culture, but their hands were filthy both before and after washing.

So 'Rule 1', learn to wash your hands properly and then teach any relatives and friends, especially children, to do so!

- Inflammation

The term Inflammation is broad and not precise, but it always involves activation of the immune system and cell division. 'Normal' or 'acute' inflammation is the body's response to an injury or infection and as such, it usually promotes healing.

However, quite frequently, the immune system seems to become 'over-zealous' and this can result in autoimmunity. The mechanisms surrounding this are poorly understood, nevertheless, it is clear that autoimmunity is increasing by 3-12% per year (depending on type of disease and region of the world) and there is little doubt that like cancer, at least some aspects of autoimmunity are also caused by environmental 'pollution' and 'toxins'.

In contrast, chronic inflammation is greatly increased by ageing[ii] and one if not the greatest cause of age-related inflammation is cells reaching their **telomere limit**.

Other causes of inflammation are:

- Having high levels of growth promoting hormones, metabolic substances, or chemicals (from drugs and toxins) in the body.
- Having low levels of physical activity.
- Experiencing chronic stress [iii].
- Having a BMI at or above 30 (<u>i.e. being obese</u>), especially when excess weight is deep within your belly – also called visceral fat.
- An imbalance of healthy and unhealthy microbes in your gut (dysbiosis).
- Regularly eating foods that cause inflammation, such as foods high in trans fats or salt.
- Disrupted sleep and disrupted circadian rhythms.

- Exposure to toxins, including air pollution, hazardous waste and industrial chemicals.
- Using tobacco products.
- Regularly drinking too much alcohol.

Stage 3 - Progression

In almost every malignant tumour, there are masses of genetic changes. To get to this stage the cells have undergone an evolution where the changes that give the most unrelenting growth advantage have been selected. The malignant cancer cell has a remarkable number of changes, some of which are probably produced by the cancer growth process itself.

Telomeres and their Importance in Cancer

In 1961 a scientist called Hayflick showed that normal cells have a built in "clock" that determines the number of times the cell can divide. He discovered this from growing cells in culture and observing that cells taken from an embryo would grow for many more cell generations than those taken from a baby. A baby's cells would grow for longer than those of a child and a child longer than an adult.

Sometime before this demonstration, cytogeneticists realised that the ends of chromosomes had special properties that set them apart from broken ends. These scientists observed that when chromosomes were *broken by radiation or chemicals* the broken ends would always join up or mend. They described this as being "sticky". In contrast, under normal circumstances the ends of chromosomes did not have any tendency to join up with other ends! The scientists thus assumed that the ends had a special structure, and they called the special ends "telomeres".

Once (the then new) DNA technology provided suitable techniques, research showed that the telomeres did indeed have a special structure.

In general, once a cell has become 'differentiated' (i.e. it's role or fate has been defined), its chromosomes can no longer replicate any part of the telomeres. Furthermore, each subsequent cell division shortens the telomeres by a tiny amount.

However, although the ability for cells to re-grow telomeres is lost in the process of differentiation, there are some exceptions. There is a 'class' of cells called *stem cells* in which telomeres are preserved. Stem cells can be regarded as a reservoir of cells in very early stages of differentiation that can be stimulated to form new adult cells. Not surprisingly they are very common in the bone marrow where new blood cells are regularly formed.

But, for most cells, their capacity to divide finishes once that cells' telomeres are shortened to a point known as the 'telomere limit'. Recent research has shown that this point occurs when the telomere is too short for the TRF2 protein to arrange the chromosome to form a telomere loop!

The end of the Line

Hayflick observed that in the last stages of a cultured cell's life, the cell makes many errors of division.

This tendency for cells to make errors in cell division has also been found to occur in the cells of people as they age, and their telomeres become shortened.

Ultimately, reduction in telomere length makes it difficult for chromosomes to attach to the spindle. Although chromosomes attach to the division spindle at the centromere (or kinetochore) constriction, the telomeres usually form special attachments near the nuclear membrane that play an important role in proper chromosome alignment in cell division.

Shortening of the telomeres inhibits proper attachment and the chromosomes are likely to make errors of division in the last cell cycles. Ultimately, the cells can no longer divide.

Should the cell 'somehow' divide after it has reached its telomere limit, the deleted telomere can become a *'sticky end'*. Such chromosomes can attach to one another at the ends and the long chromosomes formed from the combination (or translocation) of these often have more than one centromere (celled dicentric or polycentric), which leads to further problems at division and the generation of yet more abnormal chromosomes.

It is usual for cancer cells have a small amount of telomerase activity that is just enough to perpetuate cell division and allow these types of very abnormal chromosomes to form. Further division of these abnormal chromosomes expand the cancer.

The chromosomes of so-called 'solid tumours' have rarely been studied because of the technical difficulty in doing so. However, whenever they have been studied there are usually masses of chromosomal changes and cells with a wide range of differing numbers of chromosomes. All cellular controls have been lost!

In a nutshell

Put simply, a normal cell has a limited capacity to divide that is determined by its telomere length. Once the cell lineage has gone through a certain number of divisions the telomere will shorten to the point where:

a) If that cell divides, the chromosomes are extremely likely to make errors in cell division.

b) If that cell divides, telomeres may become 'sticky' and fuse with the ends of other chromosomes.

c) Fused chromosomes usually break during subsequent cell divisions and generate many more abnormalities.

Any of these conditions provide the opportunity for the selection of combinations of genes that promote malignancy.

An inevitable consequence of unbridled cell division

The tragedy is that rapid reduction in telomere length is an inevitable consequence of unbridled cell division. Thus, once a cell slips the control that stops it from dividing, the chance of malignancy is extremely high.

Benign tumour cells, like normal cells, also reduce their telomeres at every cell division. Furthermore, because benign tumours usually continue to divide, they reach the stage of minimal telomeres and potential genetic instability much faster than any normal cells and so are likely to become malignant if not suppressed.

The first major rule for cancer prevention is to reduce all unnecessary occasions of cell division.

Other Factors that may contribute to Initiation and/or Tumour Progression

Aneuploidy and polyploidy are the names given to cells having the wrong number of chromosomes. *Polyploidy* is when there are multiples of the correct number, whereas an aneuploid cell has either more, or less, chromosomes than the normal number of 46. *Aneuploidy* occurs when cell division is poorly controlled. This can be induced experimentally in several ways and studies of my colleagues and I, and those of other international studies suggest that this probably happens in the body as well.

The following are some of the key factors that disturb or "deregulate" cell division so that the cell makes errors in division.

Imbalances in pH (acid-alkaline balance).

Cells in cultures that have poor *pH control* are very prone to making errors in division. There is no reason why this would not also occur *in vivo*. The body should be slightly alkaline, about pH 7.3. Different components of cells have different pH, but the pH of each component is tightly regulated and is critical to optimal function.

In our own experiments we found, for example, that the optimal pH for lymphocytes (white blood cells) to divide was 7.6. When the pH was disturbed, individual chromosomes were more, or less, affected. Some of our bodies' pH control is derived from breathing and proper hydration but excess dietary sugar may lower blood pH and make it too acid[5]. Other factors that influence cellular pH include:

Dehydration: If cells have insufficient water, the pH and concentration of all intracellular elements is immediately affected. Thirst is a normal reflex to drink, but some people ignore this and, in time, even lose their ability to notice their thirst. Under ideal conditions we will all have an adequate intake of water from food and drink to not feel thirsty.

Having inadequate Oxygen intake (either through poor circulation, poor breathing, pollution, or lack of exercise) will also cause acid (low) pH and thus increase cancer risk.

Type 2 Diabetes and Renal Disease: Some extra evidence for the critical role disturbances of pH contribute to cancer risk comes from the links with health conditions that are associated with poor control of *cellular pH*. Two of these diseases that are well known and common are *Diabetes* and Renal Disease.

Type 2 Diabetes is associated with an increased risk of several cancers including liver, pancreatic, colorectal, bladder, endometrial and breast cancers.

Renal Disease is also associated with very high risks of many different cancers. The data is only available for people after the renal disease has been diagnosed and it is likely that there is also an earlier risk for at least <u>ten</u> different types of cancer! After dialysis, cancer risk increases to between ten and 80%!

Some of this high risk possibly reflects the shared causes of both cancer and renal disease, such as viral infections, but the pH link should not be overlooked.

Other lifestyle factors that increase the risk of cancer, and possibly also affect cellular pH are:

- Low levels of physical activity. This results in lower levels of Oxygen and higher levels of carbon dioxide.

- Chronic stress

- Having a BMI at or above 30 especially when excess weight is deep within your belly.

- An imbalance of healthy and unhealthy microbes in your gut (dysbiosis).

- Regularly eating foods that cause inflammation, such as foods high in trans fats or salt.

- Disrupted sleep and circadian rhythms.

- Exposure to toxins, including air pollution, hazardous waste and industrial chemicals.

- Using tobacco products.

Other Factors that directly affect Cell Division

In addition to pH, other common factors that adversely influence cell division include:

a) *Deficiencies in nutritional substances* that are critical for normal division (e.g. calcium) or DNA synthesis (e.g. folate)

b) *Ageing* – probably through reduction in fatty acid metabolism as cells reach their telomere limit as well as a reduction in the levels of our powerful antioxidant glutathione and key scavengers – the Superoxide dismutase enzymes.

c) *Exposures to toxic chemicals* and other *carcinogens* and their accumulation with time.

Stage 3 - Progression

In almost every malignant tumour, there are masses of genetic changes. To reach this stage the cell undergoes an evolution where the changes that give the most unrelenting growth advantage become selected.

The malignant cancer cell has a remarkable number of changes, some of which are probably produced by the cancer growth process itself.

The Value of Early Screening Programs

Although it is very likely that by adopting an excellent lifestyle, you can reduce your cancer risk considerably, it is also likely that you have already encountered several cancer risk factors. You should therefore take advantage of all the relevant early screening programs to ensure that if you do have a cancer, that it is detected as early as possible.

Advanced "benign" tumours or so-called *hyperplasia* can very easily progress to invasive tumours. It is important to make sure that these are regularly reviewed.

It is also extremely important to check out any suspicious lumps, pains, unusual tiredness, general malaise, or unusual bleeding. Do not let any of these conditions pass without a satisfactory explanation. Always be ready to ask for a second opinion if you feel that the first doctor has not taken enough notice of your request.

Chapter Three

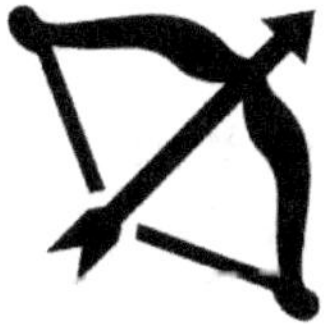

Genes that confer susceptibility to Cancer

Familial Cancer Genes

Familial cancer genes are inherited genes that confer an increased risk of developing cancer. This risk can be for cancer in general or for one specific cancer or group of related cancers. Some cancer genes confer an extremely high risk while others only confer a slightly increased risk.

How do Cancer Genes work?

The 'normal' DNA replication process itself is extremely complex and frequently generates errors. To account for this there are many checking mechanisms to make sure that the system is working to plan.

Most cancer genes disrupt the checking systems in some way - and this enables them to then escape detection.

- Several cancer genes cause defective repair of errors in DNA replication. For example, the familial colon cancer gene (MSH2) has reduced ability to repair mistakes in *DNA replication.* MSH2 and similar genes also fail to repair DNA that has been damaged in other ways.

- Several other familial cancer genes affect the body's ability to repair defects in DNA once it has occurred.

Since there are different types of DNA repair systems there are also different types of defective DNA repair genes. The genes that are known to be involved in familial breast cancer susceptibility (BRCA1 and BRCA2) each cause defective repair of double stranded breaks (i.e. a break that affects both strands of DNA simultaneously). Double strand breaks can occur spontaneously, but they also occur as a direct result of radiation, especially X-Rays.

Bloom syndrome, a rare gene that confers a high susceptibility to childhood cancer lacks a repair system that usually repairs breaks in chromosomes.

- A huge influence on an individual's susceptibility to drugs and chemical toxins is generated by a large group of genes known as the *Cytochrome P450 (CYP) genes*. This is a family of genes that generate powerful detoxification enzymes and are involved in the metabolism of 80% of prescription medications. About 57 key forms of these genes are known, with hundreds of possible genetic variations that produce a wide variety of different susceptibilities to specific toxins. It is these genes that largely influence how an individual will react to a certain toxin and is part of the explanation of why some people can get away with a lifetime of smoking cigarettes while others are highly susceptible to even second-hand smoke.

- Some critical cancer genes are involved with regulation of the cell cycle. The p53 gene (known as the guardian of the genome) is one such critical gene and perhaps our most important gene.

The p53 Gene

In its normal form the *p53* gene is known as a tumour suppressor gene because the normal product of the gene produces a protein that gives a stop signal to cell division. But when the *p53* gene is mutated, the cell containing the mutated form no longer knows *how to stop dividing.*

If a person inherits only one normally functioning copy of the *p53* gene from their parents, they are highly predisposed to cancer. Indeed, these unfortunate people usually develop several different and independent tumours in a variety of tissues in early adulthood. This rare condition of having only one normal *p53* gene is known as *Li-Fraumeni syndrome.*

Mutations in p53 are found in most tumours but in most cases the person who has the tumour is <u>not</u> born with a defective *p53* gene. Rather, the mutation of *p53* is one of the critical steps in cancer evolution within the victim's body.

Normal function of the p53 gene

The *p53* gene has been mapped to chromosome 17. In a normal cell, the *p53* gene codes for a protein that binds to a specific region of the DNA. Once this DNA protein interaction is made, this then stimulates another gene to produce a protein called *p21*. The *p21* protein itself binds to protein *cdk2*.

When the *cdk2* protein is free, it stimulates a cell to progress through cell division. However, when *p21* is complexed with *cdk2* the cell cannot pass through to the next stage of cell division.

When cells reach their Hayflick limit[6], the *p53* gene is activated and not only do cells stop dividing but fatty acid metabolism is also inhibited. Whilst this prevents cancer, the disturbances in fatty acid metabolism creates inflammation. This can be reduced by consuming (room temperature) Extra Virgin Olive Oil every day.

Mutant forms of *p53* are unable to bind DNA in an effective way and, as a result, the *p21* gene does not synthesise the *p21* protein. Because the *p21* protein has not been synthesised, the *cdk2* protein is free and cell division progresses. Cells can divide uncontrollably, and form tumours.

Although mutation or deletion of *p53* is just one possible component in the evolution of any cancer in any individual, it is usually involved. When scientists examining the DNA and/or chromosomes of cancer cells find either abnormalities of chromosome 17 or the presence of abnormal forms of *p53*, they predict a poor prognosis for the patient.

Familial mutations in the p53 gene

The following discussion should give you some idea of the relative risks conferred by a couple of different types of cancer genes.

People with the rare *Li Fraumeni syndrome* are born with a defective p53 gene in *every* cell of their body (as well as one normal gene). They are destined to get many tumours because it only takes one aberrant cell division in which *any* cell loses/deletes the chromosome 17 that carries the normal gene for cancer to commence. Once the normal chromosome 17 is lost, the block to unlimited cell division is removed and cancer can start.

In contrast, a person who carries one defective DNA repair gene (such as *MSH2* or *BRCA*) probably has about half the normal capacity to repair a DNA lesion. If such a person is exposed to a mutagen that alters the genetic sequence of a *p53* gene in one cell and this is not adequately repaired, then the individual has *one* cell with defective *p53* gene. That one cell will not necessarily cause a problem. That defective cell would need to divide as well as to lose the chromosome carrying the normal gene for unlimited division to commence.

Certainly, defective repair genes will also inhibit the ability to repair any DNA damage and damage to many other genes other than *p53* can increase the chance of cancer developing. Nevertheless, although having a defective repair gene will put someone at very much greater risk than someone with only normal repair genes, it is still a long cellular evolutionary process before a cancer becomes established.

Apart from relatively few individuals who have rare syndromes, all other cancer families share the same pathway to cancer as people without known cancer genes. People with familial cancer genes are certainly at higher risk of getting cancer than normal and so need to be more vigilant. However, the steps to cancer prevention are essentially the same for everyone.

Chapter Four

Changes in DNA and

Chromosomes that cause Cancer

Mutation

A mutation is any change in one or more elements of the genetic code of a gene. This change may or may not alter the function of the gene and so is sometimes 'benign'.

The Elements of the Genetic Code

The code of a gene is composed of triplets of the various combinations of the four nucleotide bases, adenine (A), guanine (G), cytosine (C) and thymine (T). Examples of triplets are AAT, GCC, ATG, etc.

The DNA molecule has two strands that are complementary to one another. Whenever there is an adenine in one strand, the complementary strand has a thymine and whenever one strand has a cytosine, the complementary strand has a guanine.

Protein Synthesis

The major role of the DNA code is to provide the blueprint for each protein that the body manufactures. At the beginning of protein synthesis, a gene sequence (DNA) is copied essentially unchanged into an RNA template. The only difference between an RNA and DNA sequence is that whenever a T (thymine) is incorporated in DNA this is replaced by a U (uracil) in the RNA.

The protein is then assembled alongside the RNA template. It is assembled as a structure called a peptide and several peptides will later combine to form the 3-dimensional complex form of the protein.

Only one strand of the DNA is translated into RNA. This strand is called the "sense strand".

The triplet code: Each triplet of bases is a code for either an amino acid to be added to the growing peptide chain or for a message "start replicating" or "stop here".

However, because there are 64 triplet combinations (known as codons), and only 20 amino acids that are used to make proteins, there is considerable 'redundancy'. For example, each of the following 'triplets of bases' codes for the amino acid *arginine*: CGU, CGC, CGA, CGG, AGA, AGG.

Tryptophan is the only amino acid that is coded by a single codon and the code is UGG.

Two triplets code for a *starting point*: They are AUG and GUG and there are three codons for a *stop*, namely UAG, UGA, UAA.

Gene Mutation

Several possible mistakes at the single gene level can cause an alteration in the code. During DNA synthesis, the wrong base might be incorporated, or one might be omitted. This can sometimes occur spontaneously, due to the occasional inaccuracy of the enzymes polymerising the DNA. However, errors also occur frequently in the process of repairing damage that has been caused by mutagens.

The following are common types of single gene mutations:

1. *Single Base Substitution*

Because of the redundancy of the code, many errors of single base substitution have no discernible effect. However, some wrong substitutions will code for a stop codon and any stop codon will immediately terminate the synthesis of a peptide.

Mutations that lead to the generation of an incorrect stop codon always generate a non-functional gene product.

In contrast, those that lead to the substitution of an incorrect amino acid have variable consequences, depending on the individual substitution and the region of the protein in which the substitution occurs.

There are many common inheritable mutations that involve a single base substitution.

2.   Frame Shift Mutations

When DNA synthesis or repair errors lead to a failure to incorporate a base, at the time of protein synthesis the whole reading structure moves along (or 'frame-shifts') one base from the point of error. Since the enzyme reads along the bases in one direction, every triplet after the error, will be incorrect.

It is easy to see that such an error will have a dramatic effect if it is not corrected. Frame shift mutations that are not corrected within a few bases will almost always produce a non-functional protein.

Frame-shift mutations usually occur because of strand slippage and mispairing during DNA replication. This mispairing tends to occur most frequently within runs of one nucleotide (e.g. TTTTTTTT).

Following strand slippage, the strands can re-join and repair if one or more base pairs bulge out. The mismatch is then restricted to the bulged area and the downstream nucleotides can correctly base pair. In these cases, the mutation can be corrected in the new sequence that is created in the next round of replication.

Nevertheless, this will usually produce one daughter DNA molecule with the frame- shift mutation and one daughter with the wild-type (correct) sequence.

DNA Repair Mechanisms

There are several enzyme systems in the cell that correct damage to DNA. Some of these are specific for one type of damage while others can repair a range of mutation types. These systems also differ in the degree to which they can restore the original wild-type sequence. Unfortunately, many of the repair systems *themselves induce mutations*!

Four of the best described types of repair systems are described here but there are others. Each plays a protective role and deficiencies in any one of them increases the risk for cancer.

- *Photoreactivation System (eliminated in mammals)*

Thymine dimers are a specific type of bond that is created between near-by thymidine bases when they are exposed to shorter wave- length UV. Dimers cross link the DNA and cause considerable problems if they are not repaired.

Photoreactivation utilises longer wavelength (near) UV light as well as an enzyme system to repair thymine dimers. Photoreactivation is error-free because it merely breaks the thymine dimer and restores the wild-type sequence. It is used extensively by plants, but the mechanism has been eliminated in mammals.

- *Dimer Excision Repair*

Excision repair also works on base dimers. It is much less efficient than photoreactivation and involves cutting the DNA molecule near the dimer, followed by the action of an enzyme (polar polymerase) that cuts out the thymine dimer whilst simultaneously synthesising an appropriate matching strand.

This repair system works well in cells that are not replicating.

- *Recombination repair (or post-replication repair)*

This repair mechanism works at the level of the chromosome. It repairs damage by a DNA strand exchange from the other daughter chromatid. Since it involves homologous recombination, it is largely error-free.

This type of repair can be easily visualised, and each repair point is known as a sister chromatid exchange (see below).

Figure: Sister Chromatid Exchange.

The cell on the left is taken from a normal person and the cell on the right is taken from a person with the rare genetic condition Bloom Syndrome. Bloom syndrome lacks the enzyme system RecQ helicase, which is involved in maintaining chromosome integrity. In this preparation, we have used a technique to make one chromatid dark and the other light. In the absence of an exchange, the whole chromatid will be either light or dark. Each change from dark to light is known as a

Sister Chromatid Exchange (SCE). It is easy to see that SCE frequency is low in the normal cell but high in the cell from the person with Bloom Syndrome.

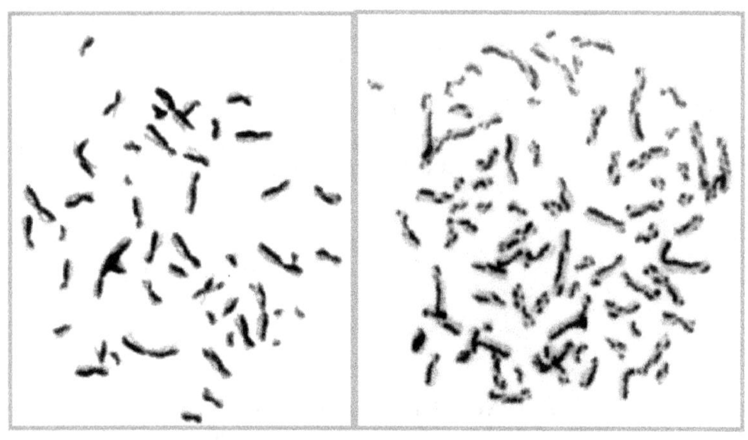

This repair system allows the identification and excision of single aberrant bases. It identifies any pair that is not perfectly matched. The aberrations may be due to the spontaneous modification of normal bases, but they also frequently caused by chemical modification.

Chromosomes and chromosome damage

Chromosomes are relatively large structures that contain spirals of DNA intertwined with protein. They vary in length at different times of the cell cycle depending on how tightly the DNA and protein are entwined. At metaphase, the stage when they are usually visualised under the microscope, the smallest chromosomes are about 1 micron long.

The relative sizes of the different chromosomes are constant, and each chromosome is recognised by its size, shape, and banding pattern. The banding pattern itself is produced (for visualisation) by various dyes, enzymic and chemical treatments but the patterns reflect the specific bases composition of the underlying DNA.

Human chromosomes are numbered from 1 to 22 (largest to smallest) plus two sex chromosomes X and Y.

Every normal <u>female</u> has a pair of each of the autosomes (1 to 22) and two X chromosomes. A normal <u>male</u>, in contrast, has a pair of each of the autosomes plus one X and one Y chromosome.

The Human Genome project established that the largest chromosome 1 has 218,712,898 DNA base pairs and the smallest chromosome 21 (actually, slightly smaller than chromosome 22 – a historical mistake in sizing) has 33,924,742 DNA base pairs.

Chromosome 22 has slightly more base pairs than chromosome 21, at 34,352. Nevertheless, in the case of chromosome 21, these nearly 34 million bases represent only about 225 functional genes in comparison to a similar number of bases representing 545 genes on chromosome 22.

Cytogeneticists, scientists who study chromosomes, might not be as surprised by this difference as the students of DNA. It has long been known that regions of chromosomes that are pale stained with Giemsa banding are particularly rich in genetic information and chromosome 21 is paler than most.

Regions that are stained darkly are often more variable in size and often contain repeated sequences of DNA that have a *regulatory* rather than an information role.

Mutation at the level of Chromosomes

There are two major types of chromosomal abnormalities, namely changes in chromosome number and changes in structure. Both types play a critical role in the initiation and progression of cancer.

Every cell should only have two copies of each autosome and a pair of sex chromosomes. This normal condition is called being diploid and is written as 2n = 46, XX (normal female), or 2n = 46, XY (normal male).

When there is one extra chromosome, i.e. three copies of one chromosome, this is described as trisomy. A cell that has 47 chromosomes, e.g. 2n = 47, XX, +21 (trisomy 21), is said to be *trisomic*. However, if there is an extra copy of every chromosome, the cell is said to be *triploid,* e.g. 3n = 69, XXY. A loss of one chromosome is called monosomy, e.g. 2n = 45, XX, -9, and a doubling of all chromosomes is called a tetraploid, e.g. 92, XXYY.

Changes in Chromosome Structure

Changes in chromosome structure occur when one or more breaks are repaired. The breaks commonly occur after exposure to *radiation* or a *toxic chemical* although they can also occur because of *severe nutritional deficiencies*.

The next series of figures illustrate some of the common outcomes of chromosomal breakage. In each case, two "normal" chromosomes are shown on the left-hand side of the diagram.

Figure: This figure depicts two normal chromosomes on the left and the positions of three breaks in the chromosomes on the right.

After breaks have occurred, there are several possible options. The first and possibly most

The initial break or breaks:

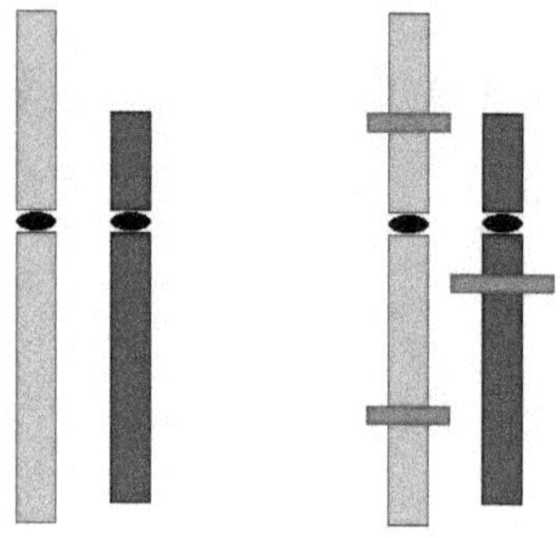

common is that the breaks can repair back to normal or near normal. There could be some mutation in the genes at the break points, but all would appear normal when looking down a microscope at the chromosome.

Rearrangements at the chromosomal level have far greater ramifications than changes at the single gene level because many genes are involved simultaneously. But nevertheless, there are still several options.

Option 1: The breaks repair back to normal.

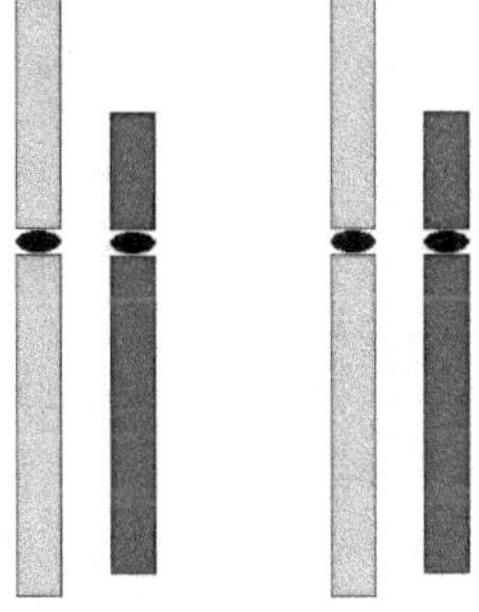

Option 2: Insertions or inversions might occur. These are called stable rearrangements because the resultant rearranged chromosomes each have a single centromere and should be able to divide normally.

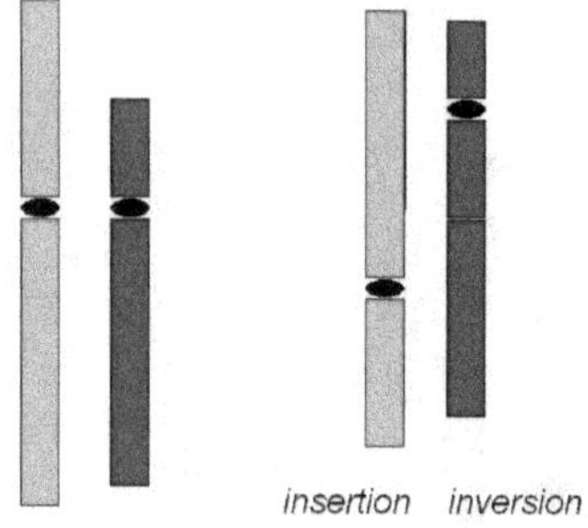

Figure: Translocations (an exchange of chromosomal material) are probably the most common type of structural exchange. Translocations, insertions, and inversions all lead to a stable chromosome form that can divide normally in all subsequent cell divisions. During the structural exchange and repair, one or many genes

might be altered. Also, there are often problems caused by change in position itself. A gene might be moved next to another gene that will change its function or expression.

 A key example of this is the 'well known' **Philadelphia (or Ph' chromosome)**. This truncated chromosome 22 was the first 'cancer chromosome' to be recognised and this finding was published in 1960! Decades later, it was shown that the Ph' chromosome resulted from a translocation between chromosomes 9 and 22 and that this involved two genes BCR and ABL1. The upregulation of tyrosine kinase that results significantly disrupts cellular 'signalling' and causes chronic myeloid leukemia (CML) as well as some cases of acute lymphatic leukemia (ALL) and acute myeloid leukemia (AML). CML accounts for 15-20% of all adult leukemias.

These aberrantly activated kinases disturb downstream signaling pathways, causing enhanced proliferation, differentiation arrest, and resistance to cell death

The following types of unstable structural rearrangements also frequently result from chromosome breakage. These forms are called unstable because they do not have the normal structure of one centromere (the black part that usually attached to the spindle machinery) and free arms.

cause translocations between chromosomes:

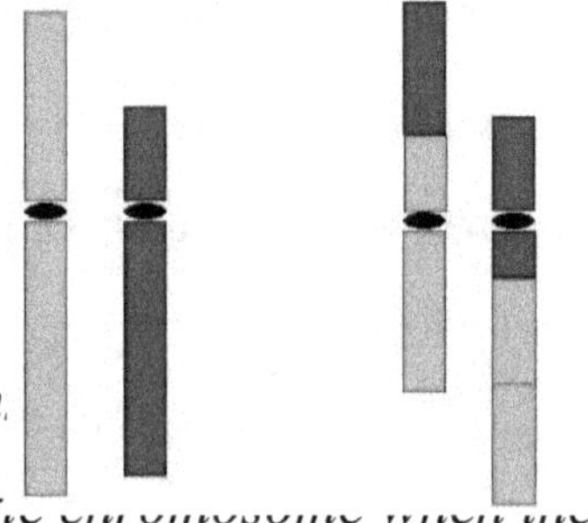

Figure: Ring ch.........rmed from two breaks in a sing...............two broken ends join up. There is often considerable loss of genetic material. Rings are reasonably unstable in division and will generate further breaks.

may cause unstable rearrangements
within chromosomes:

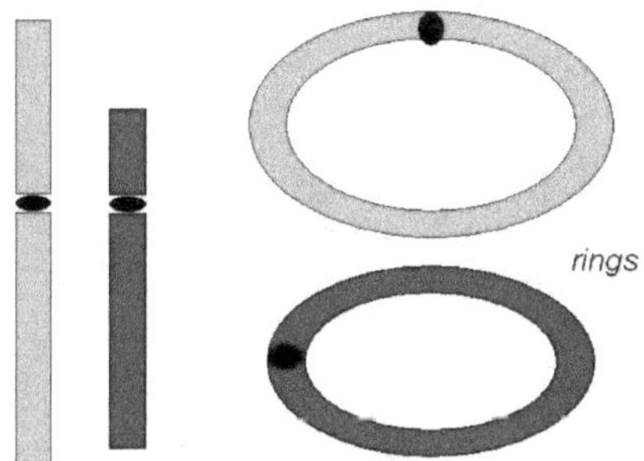

Figure: Dicentric chromosomes are also frequently seen after chromosome breakage. Since they are easy to observe they have often been used to score radiation damage. When a dicentric chromosome is formed, there are usually left-over fragments and since these cannot attach to a spindle, they are lost from the next cell division.

It is easy to see that this last type of abnormality will generate very abnormal cells. Large amounts of material will be lost as fragments at the

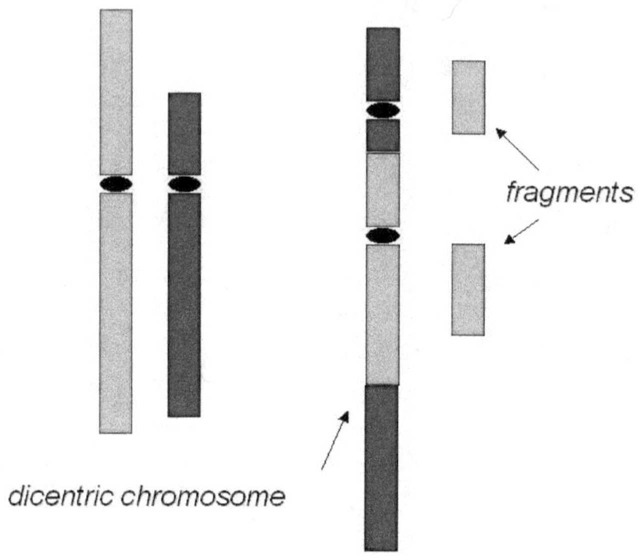

outset. But the dicentric chromosome will have difficulty dividing and lead to further complications.

A Cancer Cell showing chromosomal rearrangements

Innovative techniques, developed over many years, have allowed cytogeneticists to look at chromosomes in much the same way as I have depicted them in the diagrams. In the following Figure, each chromosome in this breast cancer cell is "painted" a different colour. There should be 46 chromosomes and two identical copies of each chromosome. But this cell possibly has no normal chromosomes remaining and it is easy to see that there are multiple rearrangements.

Figure: Example of a Breast Cancer Cell

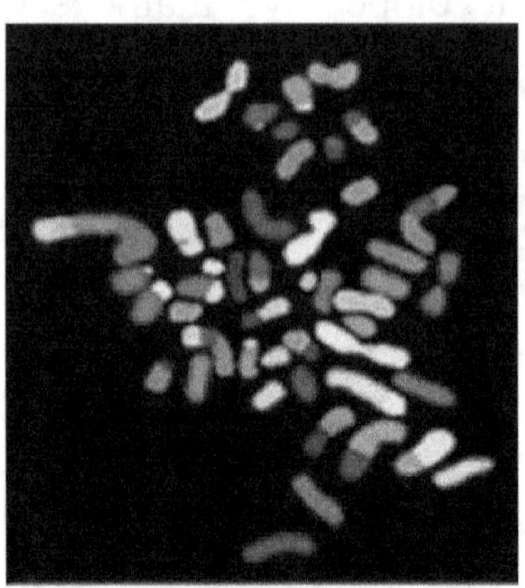

Mitosis (Cell Division) and micronuclei

Normal Mitosis

During normal mitosis, chromosomes and their DNA replicate and divide equally into two daughter cells. In the first and longest stage, when the DNA is replicating, the chromatin unravels. Some hours later, when replication is complete, the chromatin condenses, and individual chromosomes can be identified.

Metaphase: condensed chromosomes have attached to the spindle fibres. Each chromosome should be attached to the spindle at its centromere.

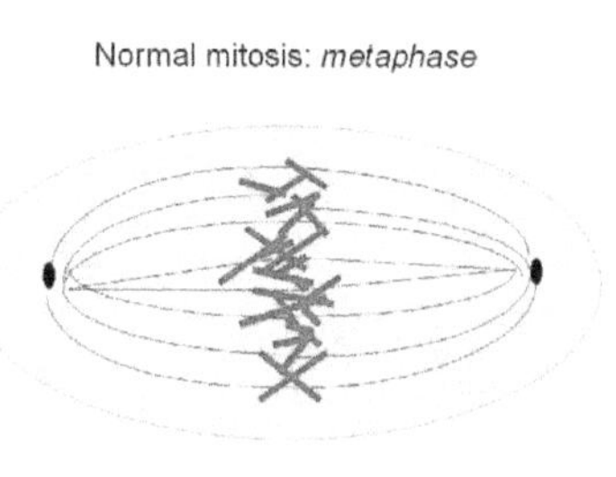

Normal mitosis: *metaphase*

Anaphase A - in which the chromosomes are repelled at the centromeres and move towards the poles.

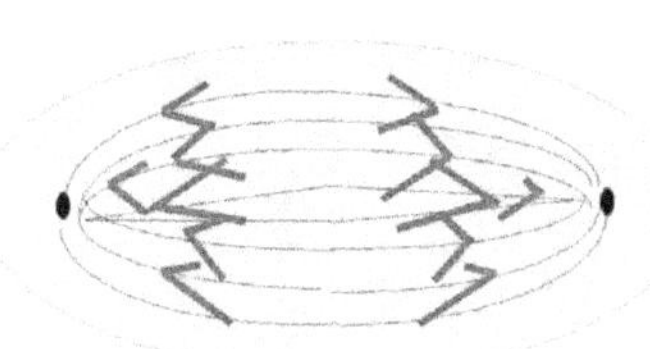

Normal mitosis: *anaphase A*

Anaphase B - in which the poles move apart, and the spindle elongates.	Normal mitosis: *anaphase B*
Telophase in which the chromosomes reach the poles	Normal mitosis: *Telophase*
Cytokinesis in which a cell plate is laid down and the two daughter cells become separate entities.	

Spindle Arrest

Under very adverse conditions, the spindle does not form. In this case the replicated chromosomes cannot move apart. After some time, the nuclear membrane reforms but the chromosome number is now double. The new cell has 92 chromosomes instead of 46.

Abnormal Spindles

Under certain (usually) pathological conditions a Unipolar or Multipolar spindle is formed. Multipolar spindles can be formed whenever the timing of cell division and chromosome replication lose their normal synchrony. Each type of spindle produces only abnormal cell progeny.

Chromosome and DNA analyses: Estimating genetic damage and aneuploidy

During the years when most of the research on mechanisms of DNA and chromosome damage were undertaken, most of the analyses were performed by experts looking at slides under the microscope. Although this is still done in some laboratories, much of this analysis is now undertaken by more automated microscopical and/or DNA techniques. These modern sophisticated techniques rely on the knowledge that was gained by painstaking microscopic analysis and, although they are much more automated and thus faster, current techniques do not always give the same detailed insight as the earlier analyses. However, they can analyse many more cells simultaneously.

Regardless of technique, geneticists regularly analyse the chromosomes and/or DNA of leukemia and estimate the extent of genetic change. From these analyses it is usually possible to define the type of leukemia and its likely prognosis.

Micronucleus analysis

Micronuclei (single – micronucleus) are small membrane bound organelles that is each a tiny nucleus. Each micronucleus contains either one or more whole chromosomes or broken bits of a chromosome. They are formed as a product of either errors in cell division, where chromosomes have failed to attach to the spindle and divide normally or a 'clastogenic' – chromosome breakage – event.

Although analysing micronuclei is not nearly as precise as analysing individual chromosomes, because it assesses large numbers of cells, it is a better measure of toxic exposures. Analysts also require far less training.

The Figure below depicts the rates of micronucleus (MN) formation by age. Over several decades, Dr Michael Fenech (CSIRO Adelaide) has introduced several refinements to the micronucleus test so that it has become much more precise and more specific. He and others have established international data sets so that very soon we hope that the test will be implemented internationally to test the safety of chemical products.

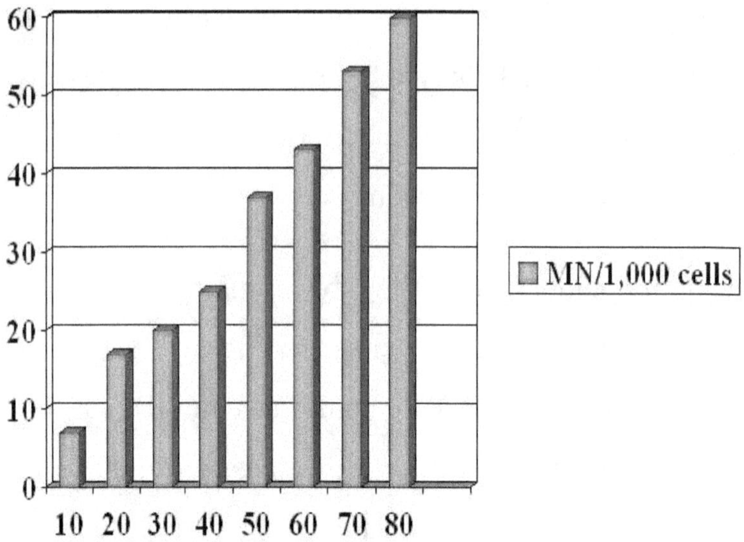

Figure: Rate of MN formation (vertical axis) with age (horizontal axis). This includes MN carrying chromosome fragments and those carrying whole chromosomes.

It is an extremely useful technique because it is simple to conduct and allows rapid evaluation of large numbers of cells and can be applied in many different situations to answer a variety of different scientific questions.

Chapter Five

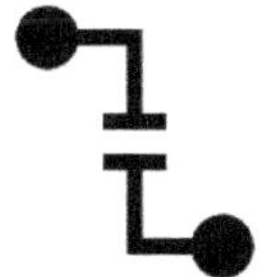

Epigenetics – yet another layer of complexity

How can development from an egg be explained?

A completely different field of research initiated the concept of *Epigenetics*. Initially the concept was invented by Conrad Waddington in 1942 in a field now known as *Developmental Genetics*. Waddington and others were striving to understand *how* the *same* chromosomes and genes could lead to such different outcomes in different cells and tissues?

This question led to the discovery of the first type of epigenetic control, known as DNA methylation. Within the chromosomes, clusters of CG (cytosine, guanine base pairs) undergo a subtle chemical change called methylation and these groups of modified base pairs are clustered together in parts of genes known as *CpG Islands*. These CpG Islands, between about 500 and 1500 base pairs long, are now known to play a critical role in suppressing an individual gene and thereby controlling or inhibiting its expression in a tissue. In essence they lock a gene in the "off" position.

Methylation can be observed under the microscope by staining cells with an immunofluorescent labelled antibody for 5-methyl cytosine. When mammalian cell preparations are observed under a fluorescent microscope, methylated bases are distributed in definite CpG sequences throughout the cells. They are not, however, found in regions with high concentrations of CpG sequences. (known as CpG islands). These islands, and other areas of high CpG content seem to play important roles in tumour suppression, (especially because they contain many tumour suppressor genes), and if they become hypermethylated, they promote cancer.

CpG island hypermethylation is a phenomenon that is important for the regulation of gene expression in cancer cells and hypermethylation of CpG islands has been described in almost every type of tumour.

Some of the key cellular pathways that are suppressed by the hypermethylation of CpG islands include **DNA repair, cell cycle regulation, apoptosis** and **cell**

adherence. Nevertheless, it is still not known to what extent hypermethylation silences tumour suppressor cells?

Histones: A second common type of epigenetic control involves the histone proteins that are part of the three-dimensional structure of chromosomes. Ever since it was discovered that histones are within chromosomes, it has been assumed that they played a part in controlling gene expression. Now, it is known that various chemical tags can modify the tightness with which the DNA is coiled around the histones and that this relaxing and tightening causes changes in the expression of the genes.

Epigenetics – in life

In general, epigenetic modifications are relatively stable and can be transferred from one cell generation to the next within an individual. But epigenetic changes do NOT change the underlying DNA and, usually, any modifications are reset in the cells that give rise to eggs and sperm and are not passed on to future generations.

There seem to be some exceptions to this where some modified DNA can be passed on through the female. Although these exceptions support the concept of imprinting, this is generally regarded as the exception rather than the rule.

And then there is RNA......!

In addition to the two types of DNA modifications defined as epigenetic control, there is still further control from so-called *non-coding* ribonucleic acid (nc) RNAs. These ncRNAs <u>may make up as much as 80% of the transcribed genome</u>. They do not code for proteins but play major regulatory roles in gene expression. The ncRNAs may play key roles in cancer, and some are now major targets for cancer therapies.

Outside cancer, dysregulation of ncRNAs possibly contribute to many if not all neurological disorders, including addiction!

Although ncRNAs differ from the classical definition of epigenetic regulators because they do not modify chromatin structure, their ability to regulate gene expression in several ways gives them many possible roles in carcinogenesis. The ncRNAs are never translated into functional proteins but are nonetheless functional.

There are two main groups, based on size: the first are short-chain non- coding RNAs (and include siRNAs, microRNAs (miRNAs), and piRNAs) and the second are longer non-coding RNA (lncRNAs).

These RNA species are a heterogeneous class of RNA transcripts and play many key roles in processes as important as development and tissue differentiation. One of their roles is *X-chromosome inactivation*: the process of silencing one of the X chromosomes in all the somatic cells of females. Furthermore, there is new evidence emerging that demonstrates that they play important roles in numerous important cellular processes associated with differentiation, and development.

Some lncRNAs have key regulatory roles including mRNA stability, protein translation, and protein stability. They do not just modulate gene activity in time and space, but they also regulate critical biological processes such as DNA responses to damage, DNA repair, and DNA replication.

Cancer epigenetics -

Cancer biology is extraordinarily complex because it involves an interplay between genetic and epigenetic abnormalities. Cancers are self-serving and, within every cancer, both genetic and epigenetic changes are selected to be mutually beneficial for driving the cancer's initiation and progression.

The earliest cancer research occurred before even cells were discovered! So, although the concept of

Epigenetics was coined in 1942, its critical role in cancer has only been elaborated in the last ten years.

The importance of epigenetic alterations was first elaborated in paediatric cancers, especially brain tumours. Few other genetic abnormalities were ever found in these tumours, but they were found to have abnormal epigenetic patterns.

In many other cancers, the key role of epigenetic changes has emerged from DNA sequencing studies. The collaborative international efforts to sequence the genome of thousands of human cancers have demonstrated the presence of frequent alterations in numerous epigenetic regulators. The identification of these key changes is allowing key steps to be made in more accurate diagnosis and prediction of prognosis. The next step is likely to be the design of and possible treatment with epigenetic-targeted drugs.

To make things even more complex, in some situations both 'classical' genetic changes and epigenetic changes **can have the same disease outcome**!

For example, *either* a chromosomal deletion or an epigenetic change of a specific region of chromosome 11 plays a key role in Chronic Lymphocytic Leukemia. Chronic lymphocytic leukemia (CLL) is a relatively benign leukemia that usually only affects people after middle age and progresses slowly. In this disease many lymphocytes become somewhat abnormal and cannot fight infections very effectively.

In 1983, my own laboratory worked out a way of stimulating CLL cells to grow using a mitogen called TPA (12-0-tetradecanylphorbol-13-acetate). Once we could grow the cells, we were able to examine the chromosomes, and we found that the cells from many of the patients had a deletion of part of the long arm of chromosome 11[7].

It is exciting to see now that recent DNA research has found that there is a cluster of *microRNA genes* located in this commonly deleted region of chromosome 11 and that these miRNAs are known to be epigenetically regulated.

Whilst this specific chromosomal site can be located and the biology/biochemistry of the effect of the damage is starting to be described, this research still does not identify the cause(s). So, although this understanding should help greatly with finding better treatments or even a cure, it still leaves the unanswered question of why it happens. Is it just one or more chance event in a person who lives a long life?

In Summary

There is clearly much more to be known about the changes that occur in the chromosomes and genetic machinery that allow cancer to develop. However, this overview should give you considerable insight into the complexity of cancer and why it is so insidious.

We will probably never prevent cancer, but we can reduce some of our risks. Currently some of our key actions are:

- Vaccination against known cancer-causing viruses.

- Modification of poor 'lifestyle', home and 'work practices' to reduce exposure to known carcinogens.

- Modification of diet and lifestyle to optimise our cellular pH.

- Taking action to reduce extraneous CELL DIVISION.

- As you age, as advised (and explained) in my book '*Why We Age*', consume Oleic Acid daily (from either Olive oil or Sesame Oil) and consume foods that support your key enzymes *glutathione transferase* and *superoxide dismutase*.

Wishing you a healthy long life!

References

I.   Erlich P (1968) The Population Bomb. Sierra Club. Ballantine Books.

II.   Li, X., Li, C., Zhang, W *et al.* Inflammation and aging: signalling pathways and intervention therapies. *Sig Transduct Target The r***8**, 239 (2023). https://doi.org/10.1038/s41392-023-01502-8

III.   https://my.clevelandclinic.org/health/diseases/11874-stress

IV.   Ford JH & Roberts CG (1983) Chromosome displacement and spindle tubule polymerization: 1. The effect of alterations in pH on displacement frequency. Cytobios 37: 163-169

V.   Resnick LM (1992) Cellular ions in hypertension, insulin resistance, obesity, and diabetes: a unifying theme. J Am Soc Nephrol. Oct;3(4 Suppl):S78-85.

VI.   Ford, J.H. (2019) Why We Age page 23 and Chapter 4.

VII.   Callen DF & Ford JH (1983) Chromosome abnormalities in chronic lymphocytic leukemia revealed by TPA as a mitogen. Cancer Genetics & Cytogenetics 10: 87-93

www.ingramcontent.com/pod-product-compliance
Lightning Source LLC
Chambersburg PA
CBHW050804250726
48653CB00006B/2067